Contents

WELCOME   2

3-DAY DETOX RECIPES
Christin's Power Breakfast   5
Instant Pot Veggies and Starch   6
Veggie Lover's Pizza Potato   7
Banana Bread Overnight Oats   8
Mediterranean Rice   9

3-DAY DETOX FAQ   10

3-DAY DETOX GROCERY LIST   12

GREEN LIGHT CHEAT SHEET   13

FOOD AND MOOD JOURNAL   14

Welcome to your 14-Day Reboot Challenge!

We're so glad you have taken this step to catapult your health and vitality to the next level. Whether you're brand new to a plant-based diet or a long time expert who just needs a few tweaks to stay on track, you're in the right place. We have amazing resources that have proven time and time again to help people blast through plateaus and finally see the results they've been looking for.

This Starter Kit was created as a companion kit to the 14-Day Reboot Challenge online coaching program. For more info or to register for the next challenge, visit www.TheForeverDiet.org.

What you'll find inside are hard copy versions of the digital materials included with the 14-Day Reboot Challenge online coaching program. Everything is explained in full detail inside the coaching program. The Food and Mood Journal is a key tool for accountability. You'll be sharing your daily journal with your accountability partner. Take a few minutes every morning to plan ahead for the day, track your food and mood throughout the day, and review at the end of the day to record how well you did hitting your targets.

We kick off the program with a 3-Day Detox to give your body a true reboot! This is a chance for you to not even think about your food for a change. Just make these detox recipes and enjoy them! This detox was created almost accidentally! Every time I have weekend visitors to our house, we would get a phone call Monday morning with an excited guest who had lost weight just by visiting! See, they would eat the food I put in front of them, and they would lose weight without even trying! That's what the 3-Day Detox can be for you - just make the food I would put in front of you if you came to visit. This will help get you through the worst of the withdrawl symptoms from your formerly rich diet, and will help you reset to actually enjoy a health-promoting diet.

I have included the recipes as well as a grocery list to prepare these recipes. Compare against what you have at home and simply cross off things you probably already have, like cinnamon and rolled oats. Purchase what you need, take some time to cook everything all at once, and you'll be ready to roll for Day 1!

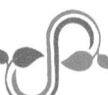

You'll also find in the Starter Kit a handy resource called the Green Light Cheat Sheet. This is a visual representation of our dietary recommendations. The program is about MUCH more than the food, of course, but this spells out for you what our food recommendations are.

If you have questions at any time, please reach out for help! Reach for your accountability partner, post in the private accountability group, or email me at Chris@TheForeverDiet.org.

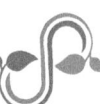

The ForeverDiet

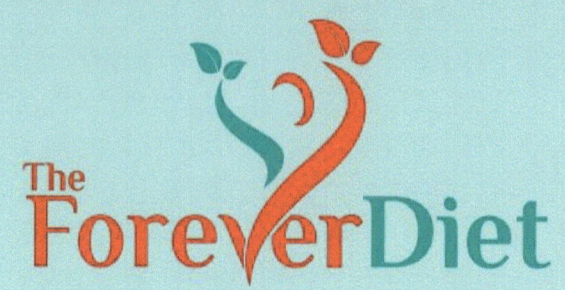

3-DAY DETOX

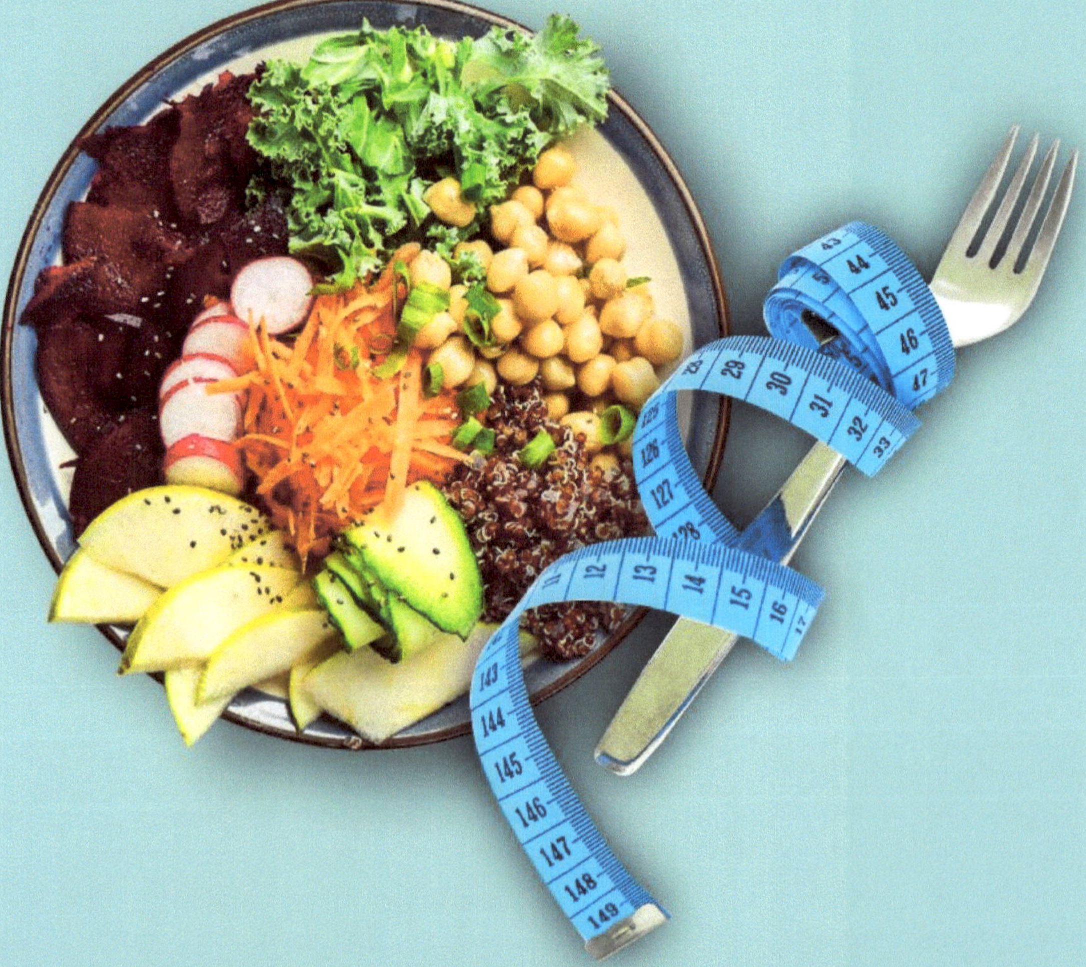

By Christin Bummer

Christin's Power Breakfast

🕐 Prep time: 08 minutes   🍲 Cook time: N/A   🍴 Yield: 4 Servings

This is my favorite post-workout breakfast. It's packed with protein and heart healthy nutrients, with just enough sweetness to make it delicious.

🧺 Ingredients:

- ❖ 32 oz frozen chopped spinach
- ❖ 16 oz crushed pineapple in juice
- ❖ 3 c cooked chickpeas (30 oz canned)
- ❖ ½ - 1 Tbsp cinnamon

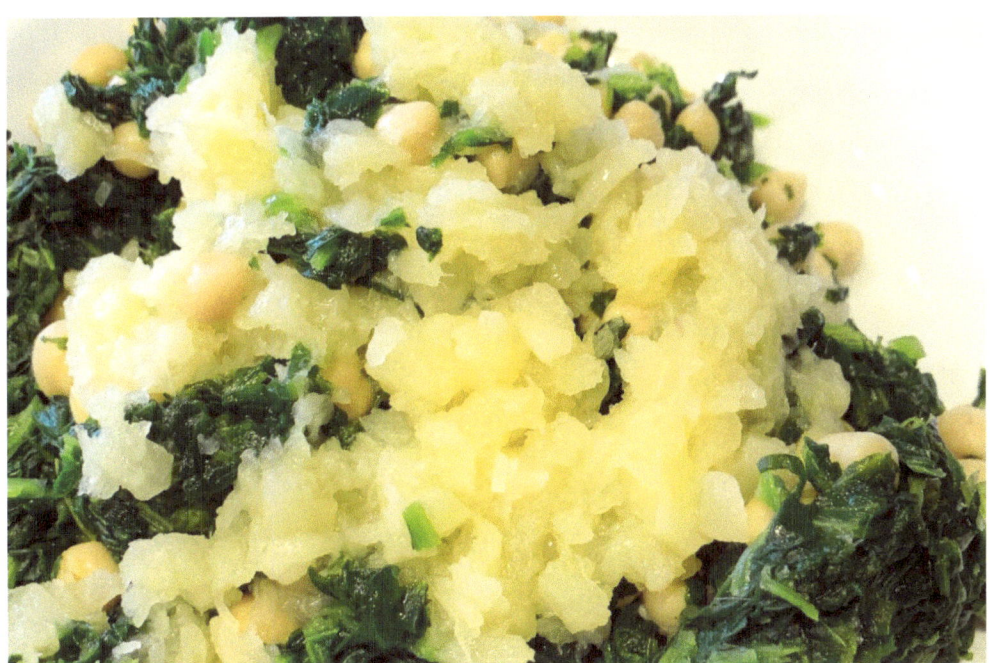

👤 Instructions:

Thaw spinach in colander under hot water. Squeeze excess water. Drain and rinse chickpeas. Transfer to mixing bowl. Add pineapple and cinnamon and stir with a fork. Enjoy!

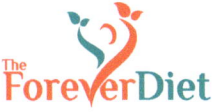

Instant Pot Veggies and Starch

 Prep time: 01 minutes   Cook time: Varies   Serving Size: Unlimited

Sometimes we make cooking WAY harder than it needs to be. 75% of our meals in a week look something like this! It's nice to have the fun recipes, but it's also very freeing to keep it simple and realistic.

Ingredients:

- ❖ your favorite veggies
- ❖ your favorite starches

Instructions:

Steam your favorite veggies, potatoes, and squash in the Instant Pot according to the following timetables. Add 1 cup of water and use the natural release. Your texture preferences may vary, but this is a general guide:

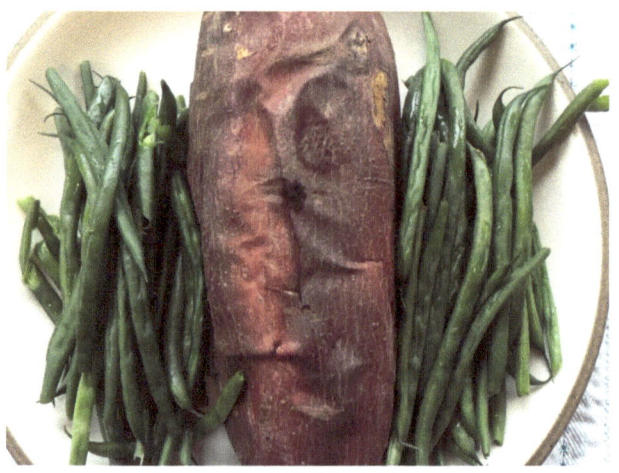

STARCHES
1 c of water, steamer rack,
natural release

Potatoes *(cut into medium chunks)*: 4-5 mins
Potatoes (whole): 8-12 mins depending on size
Sweet Potatoes (whole): 10-15 mins depending on size
Acorn squash (whole): 7-8 mins
Butternut squash (whole): 25 mins
Kabocha squash (whole): 8-10 mins
Spaghetti squash (whole): 6-8 mins

VEGGIES
1 c of water,
QUICK release

Brussels Sprouts: 3 min (whole)

Green Beans: 1 min

Carrots: 1 min

Broccoli: 0 min

Cauliflower: 0 min

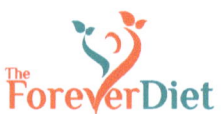

Veggie Lover's Pizza Potato

Prep time: 10 minutes   Cook time: 50 minutes   Yield: 3-4 servings

I once was at an Italian restaurant that had nothing but a salad on the menu that would have been compliant. But, they had baked potatoes and pizza toppings. And voila! The Pizza Potato was born.

Ingredients:

- 4-6 yukon gold potatoes, baked
- 2 bell peppers, diced
- 2 red onions, diced
- 8 oz mushrooms, sliced
- 2 c broccoli, chopped
- 1 tsp garlic powder

- 1 tsp onion powder
- oil-free hummus
- 8 oz tomato paste
- oil-free sun-dried tomatoes *(optional)*
- pineapple *(optional)*
- crushed red pepper

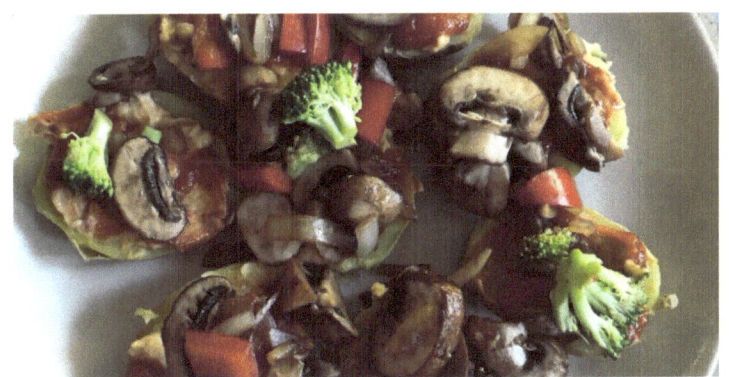

Instructions:

Preheat oven to 375 degrees. Bake potatoes 375 degrees for 45-50 minutes. Chop bell peppers, onions, mushrooms, and broccoli. Sprinkle with garlic and onion powder, then roast in the same oven 20-25 minutes. Split open potatoes, smash gently with a fork to form a flat surface. Spread with hummus and tomato paste, then top with bell peppers, red onions, mushrooms, broccoli, and spices. For more pizazz, add sun-dried tomatoes and/or pineapple, or your other favorite veggies. Return to oven for 5 minutes.

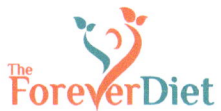

Banana Bread Overnight Oats

🕐 Prep time: 2 minutes   🍲 Refrigerate: Overnight   🍴 Yield: 4 servings

Make a batch or two of this oatmeal and you'll have oatmeal ready to grab and go! No more babysitting oats over the stovetop or reheating a gummy mess the next day. This is great for those transitioning away from a standard american breakfast. If you're already used to a savory breakfast, you may wish to use this as a dessert recipe instead!

🧺 Ingredients:

- 2 c rolled oats
- 2 ripe bananas, mashed
- 2 c unsweetened non-dairy milk
- 2 tsp cinnamom
- 1 tsp cardamon

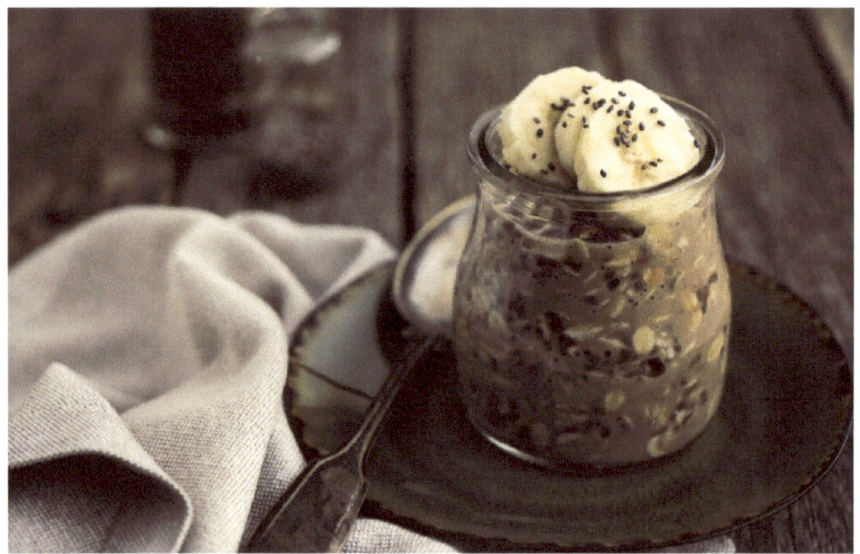

👤 Instructions:

Add all ingredients to a mixing bowl, combine. Store in refrigerator overnight. Stir and serve warm or cold. Serve plain or top with fresh berries. If oats aren't your thing, or if you want a TRULY fool-proof whole-grain version, you can try this with cooked rice or quinoa....

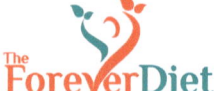

Mediterranean Rice

Prep time: 10 minutes | 20 minutes, then quick release | Yield: 6-8 servings

Move over South Beach Diet, this dish will run circles around you! Enjoy all the flavors of the Mediterranean Rice without all of the calories! The original recipe was formulated for the Instant Pot, but a stovetop version is shown below.

Ingredients:

- 1 c sweet onion, diced
- 2 c sweet potato, diced
- 2 Tbsp Kirkland's No-Salt Seasoning or Benson's Table Tasty
- 1 tsp garlic powder
- 1 tsp celery seed
- ½ tsp cinnamon
- 1 c dried green or brown lentils
- 1 ½ c brown jasmine rice
- ½ c oil-free sun-dried tomatoes, chopped
- 15 oz can fire roasted diced tomatoes
- ½ c red or white quinoa
- 6 c water

Instructions:

Instant Pot: Put all ingredients into and Instant Pot. Cook for 20 minutes, then quick release.

Stovetop: Saute onion in a large nonstick soup pot for 3-5 minutes. Add water as needed to prevent sticking. Stir in spices, potato, rice and lentils. Add remaining ingredients. Bring to a boil. Reduce heat, cover and simmer for 45-50 minutes, stirring occasionally. Add extra water (1 cup at a time) as needed to prevent sticking.

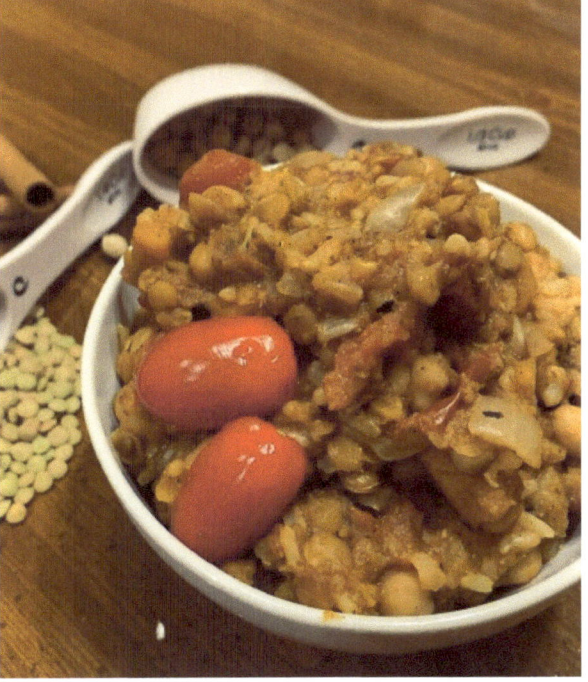

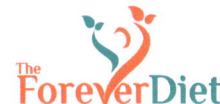

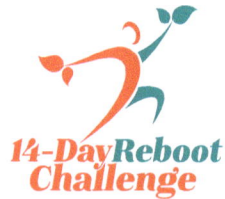

As you read in *Ditch Dieting Forever*, we're going to kick things off with a 3-Day Detox! This allows you to dive right in and start experiencing this new way of eating without wasting another minute.

I encourage you to use this opportunity to try something new. I know there are people entering this Challenge with drastically different backgrounds. Some of you have been whole food plant-based for many years. Others are dabbling with vegetarianism for the first time. Many are used to having processed, prepared, or restaurant foods make up a fairly significant portion of your diet. This is a chance to start fresh, and I urge you to take full advantage of it by going all-in rather than censoring the suggestions or doing things your own way.

I encourage you to keep an open mind. If you keep doing what you've always done, you're going to get what you've always gotten... Do your best to stick to the detox as suggested. Later in the program I'll be explaining why I've chosen these specific ingredients, I promise! There's just not time to explain all the do's and don'ts up front!

There are common questions that come up so please read these FAQ's to better understand what to expect.

💡 How much should I eat?

As much as you want! You are likely to experience some cravings and withdrawal symptoms during the initial transition to this Challenge. The most important thing is to stay on plan as much as you possibly can. I promise that the closer you stay to the plan, the simpler it is and the faster you can say good-bye to cravings. So, if you're hungry, eat! Just stick to the Detox Recipes and let the rest go.

I've put yields on the recipes to give you a ROUGH idea of how much each recipe makes (not so that you'll restrict your servings or portions). BONUS: You're likely to have leftovers to keep you covered for a few more days.

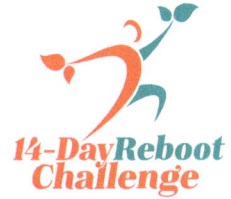

💡 What about making substitutions?

This is a tricky one. Certainly, if you have allergies or food sensitivities, you'll just make adjustments as needed. Omit any of the recipes if you need to. And remember, one of the recipes is "Instant Pot Veggies and Starch" which is a fancy way of saying – you can eat whatever steamed veggies and starch you wish (ex: potatoes, rice, quinoa, beans)!

💡 What happens after the Detox?

We'll get to that, I promise! After the first three days of video lessons, you're going to better understand the program and the reasons behind it. If you can't get more groceries mid-week, you may wish to plan to make a second round of the detox recipes. There's certainly no harm in that.

💡 What about coffee?

If you're currently drinking coffee, I wouldn't recommend ditching caffeine right now. It's often too much of a change for people during the Reboot Challenge and there are too many other critical things to focus on right now. In the meantime, consider switching to black or an unsweetened non-dairy creamer.

💡 What about snacking?

When you're hungry, eat! Whether your snack is another serving of a detox recipe, a plain potato, some fruit, or some veggies, go ahead and snack! We're not going to worry about sticking to strict mealtimes or eating according to the clock at this point in the game. A lot of those techniques have sent people down a path to troublesome yo-yo dieting. Rest assured, if you're eating food on the detox plan over the course of the next 3 days, you can let go of your concern about snacking, eating too much, etc. Again, I'll be explaining much more about this as we get going.

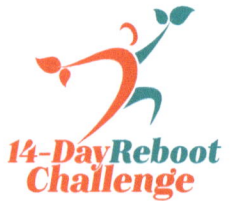

3-Day Detox FAQ
(Grocery List)

Veggies and Fruit

- [ ] 2 ripe bananas
- [ ] 1 sweet onion
- [ ] 2 sweet potatoes
- [ ] 4-6 Yukon gold potatoes
- [ ] 2 bell peppers
- [ ] 2 red onions
- [ ] 8 oz mushrooms
- [ ] 1 head broccoli

Instant Pot Veggies and Starch

- [ ] 5 lbs of favorite veggies
- [ ] More brown rice or quinoa
- [ ] favorite potatoes
- [ ]

Dry Grains + Beans

- [ ] 1 ½ c brown jasmine rice
- [ ] ½ c red or white quinoa
- [ ] 2 c rolled oats
- [ ] 1 c dried green or brown lentils

Other

- [ ] 2c non-dairy milk
- [ ] 1 c oil-free sun-dried tomatoes
- [ ] hummus (oil free if poss)
- [ ] 32 oz frozen spinach

Canned

- [ ] 16 oz crushed pineapple
- [ ] 30 oz chickpeas
- [ ] 8 oz tomato paste
- [ ] 15 oz fire-roasted diced tomatoes

Spices

- [ ] cinnamon
- [ ] cardamom
- [ ] Kirkland's No-Salt Seasoning or Benson's Table Tasty
- [ ] garlic powder
- [ ] celery seed
- [ ] onion powder
- [ ] crushed red pepper

Frozen

- [ ] 32 oz frozen spinach
- [ ]

Anytime Snacks

- [ ] any fruit you enjoy:
- [ ] Ex: apples, oranges, grapes,
- [ ] banana, watermelon, cherries, etc
- [ ] any raw veggies you enjoy:
- [ ] carrots, sugar snap peas, etc
- [ ] Herbal tea for iced tea if you wish
- [ ] Lemons for lemon water if you wish

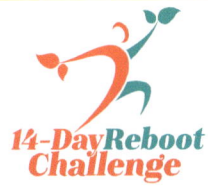

14-DayReboot Challenge

GREEN LIGHT FOODS:
No Limits! The More the Merrier

All leafy greens: Spinach, bok choy, kale, collards, romaine. cabbage, etc

All vegetables: Bell peppers, red beets, tomatoes, carrots, broccoli, cauliflower, celery, zucchini eggplant, onions, mushrooms, etc

Starches: Potatoes, sweet potatoes, squashes, plantains etc

Legumes: Lentils (all colors), chickpeas, black beans, pinto beans, kidney beans, mung beans

Whole Grains: Brown rice, quinoa, oats, millet, amaranth, etc

Fruit: Apples, oranges, plantains, strawberries, raspberries, kiwi, blueberries, grapes, blackberries, melon, cherries, bananas, and more

Preparations: Raw, steamed, boiled, roasted, or air-fried are all perfectly fine!

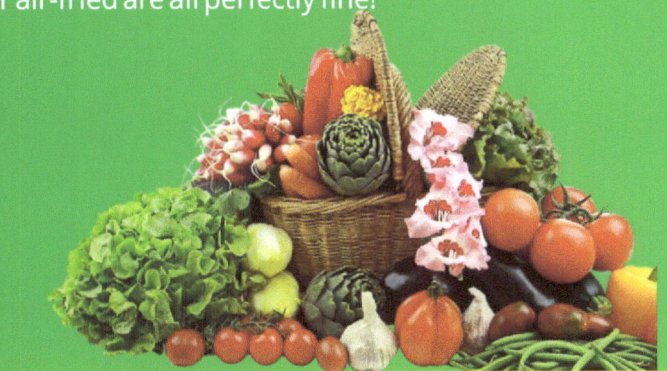

YELLOW LIGHT FOODS:

Proceed with Caution. These foods are all calorically dense.

Nuts And Nut Butters

Coconut

Seeds *(includes seed bread & crackers)*

Avocado

Dried Fruit

Tofu, Tempeh

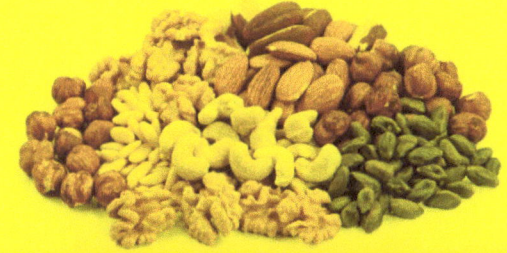

RED LIGHT FOODS:
These Foods Do Not Serve You! Stay Away!

All animal products: If it walks, flies, swims, or has a mother, let it be. That is, meat, fish, birds, eggs, or dairy.

All oils: coconut, olive, canola, vegetable, flax seed, grape seed, etc. This includes anything deep fried, cooked in oil, or with oil listed in the ingredients.

All highly processed foods: sugar, flour, alcohol, or products made with them.

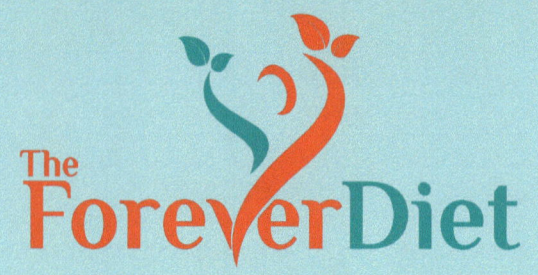

FOOD & MOOD Journal

By Christin Bummer

Congratulations! You have taken the first step in establishing new habits! Give yourself a pat on the back, and let's get started. Simply dedicate a few minutes every day to set yourself set up for success. There are three main sections on each page.

1) Each morning you will have a chance to record your sleep from the previous night, and you will take some time to think about the upcoming day. When and how can you sneak in extra movement? What challenges are coming up? Perhaps you have a work meeting, a restaurant date, or even just a day lounging around the house with your friends or family. Where are you going to face temptation and what are you going to do about it? Planning is half the battle.

Think about your tools. How can you use them to your advantage to get through those challenge-tunities?! As you get farther along in the process you'll start to recognize potential areas for triggers. Once you identify them, you can better plan ahead to overcome them. There are no mistakes, just opportunities to learn.

2) Throughout the day, record your food and beverage intake. Jot down what you ate for each meal and snack, and approximately how much (eg. A big bowl of veggies, 2 medium potatoes, and a couple kiwi). We DO NOT want you counting calories, but it's very common to UNDER-eat when you're first getting started with a whole food plant-based diet. When you record approximate amounts, you'll get better feedback from your coach and from your accountability partner.

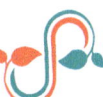

It's also important to note your moods before and after each meal, as appropriate. Are you bright-eyed and bushy-tailed or sluggish? Happy or sad? Anxious? Overcome by cravings or at ease? Starving? Bored?

Stumped for adjectives to describe your mood? Here are some more to get you started:

Elated	Motivated	Frustrated	Cheerful	Calm
Confident	Happy	Depressed	Bored	Anxious
Excited	Manic	Panicked	Stressed	Impatient
Guilty	Embarrassed	Fearful	Ashamed	Lonely
Angry	Cranky	Blissful	Sluggish	Nervous
Comfortable	Irritable	Fantastic	Healthy	At Ease

3) At the **end of each day**, take time to reflect. What went well? Not so well? What could you improve upon for next time? Having your own suggestions for improvement at the forefront of your mind will help propel you forward in your transformation. This is not a place to beat yourself up, but rather to objectively evaluate your progress and identify the most effective areas for improvement.

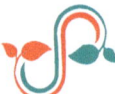

We've created the acronym PLANTS as a code word to keep you focused. You'll track these main objectives that are critical to creating your Forever Diet. Record your PLANTS progress for the day by checking the box for each target that you hit.

Here's what each stand for:

P – Planning ahead. Make sure your kitchen is stocked, and you have a plan to stay on track even if you're eating at someone else's house, at work, etc.

L – Lots of healthy food, eating and enjoying lots of healthy food, that is!

A – Activity – getting some kind of intentional activity in every day. This could be a rigorous workout 45 mins to an hour, or a gentle walk after dinner. Taking the stairs instead of the elevator or parking as far away as you can manage counts. Add activity wherever YOU can!

N – Nice – being a nice person, doing something nice for someone else, AND most importantly, being kind to yourself.

T – Thankful – being thankful, and living in gratitude will help you go far. This could mean taking a few minutes to meditate daily, or to pray if that's your thing, or just to pause and reflect.

S – Sleep – Getting lots of sleep is crucial! See if you can work

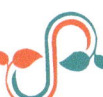

toward waking up feeling rested, without an alarm. That's when you're sleep satiated. Usually 8-9 hours is best for most people. There are NO right or wrong answers here. This is your own tracking tool and you are welcome to interpret the targets any way THAT WORKS for you. Don't fool yourself, but also don't be too hard on yourself. Got it?

There's more good news... You are NOT expected to hit every single target 100% every single day. That's not realistic and that's not necessarily even a good goal. Instead, we want you to strive for 80% success. So after you've logged 7 days, count up how many targets you hit for the week. There are 6 letters in PLANTS and 7 days of the week. That makes 42 targets total. If you've hit 33 targets or more, you've achieved the goal! If you didn't, just take a look at where you can improve. Where are you struggling? We'll walk you through a little analysis when you get there.

If you're rocking the Planning, Lots of food, and Activity, but you haven't gotten a single N for nice or a T for thankful... then that's a good area to focus on for next week! Living the good life isn't JUST about the food or rock hard abs. It's not about fitting into a skinnier casket! This program is intended to help you become the best YOU that you can be, and we know you're a nice, thankful person. At least 80% of the time!

All right, enough reading, let's get started!

Su Mo Tu We Th Fr Sa   Date:_____

Last night, I went to bed at_____, I woke up at_____, I got_____ hrs of sleep

I slept: GREAT!   Good   Not so bad   Interrupted   UGH, bad

Today I felt so thankful for:_____

_____

How and when I can be active today:_____

_____

Challenges I expect to face today:_____

_____

I plan to overcome by:_____

_____

Food & Mood

Time of day	Food and Drink	I'm Feeling.......
Wake to 8am		
8am to 10am		
10am to 12pm		
12noon to 2pm		
2pm to 4pm		
4pm to 6pm		
6pm to 8pm		
8pm to 10pm		

Targets for the Day: P L A N T S

Give yourself a check for each target: ☐ ☐ ☐ ☐ ☐ ☐

(Plan ahead, Lots of healthy food, Activity, Nice, Thankful, Sleep)

Notes and Homework Assignments:_____

_____

_____

_____

_____

_____

_____

_____

_____

_____

_____

_____

_____

_____

_____

_____

_____

_____

Tomorrow I will focus on:_____

_____

_____

Su Mo Tu We Th Fr Sa   Date:_____

Last night, I went to bed at_____, I woke up at_____, I got_____ hrs of sleep

I slept: GREAT!   Good   Not so bad   Interrupted   UGH, bad

Today I felt so thankful for:_____

_____

How and when I can be active today:_____

_____

Challenges I expect to face today:_____

_____

I plan to overcome by:_____

_____

Food & Mood

Time of day	Food and Drink	I'm Feeling.......
Wake to 8am		
8am to 10am		
10am to 12pm		
12noon to 2pm		
2pm to 4pm		
4pm to 6pm		
6pm to 8pm		
8pm to 10pm		

Targets for the Day: P L A N T S

Give yourself a check for each target: ☐ ☐ ☐ ☐ ☐ ☐

(Plan ahead, Lots of healthy food, Activity, Nice, Thankful, Sleep)

*Notes and Homework Assignments:*_____

_____

_____

_____

_____

_____

_____

_____

_____

_____

_____

_____

_____

_____

_____

_____

_____

_____

_____

*Tomorrow I will focus on:*_____

_____

_____

Su Mo Tu We Th Fr Sa   Date:_____

Last night, I went to bed at_____, I woke up at_____, I got_____ hrs of sleep

I slept: GREAT!   Good   Not so bad   Interrupted   UGH, bad

Today I felt so thankful for:_____
_____

How and when I can be active today:_____
_____

Challenges I expect to face today:_____
_____

I plan to overcome by:_____
_____

Food & Mood

Time of day	Food and Drink	I'm Feeling.......
Wake to 8am		
8am to 10am		
10am to 12pm		
12noon to 2pm		
2pm to 4pm		
4pm to 6pm		
6pm to 8pm		
8pm to 10pm		

Targets for the Day: P L A N T S

Give yourself a check for each target: ☐ ☐ ☐ ☐ ☐ ☐

(Plan ahead, Lots of healthy food, Activity, Nice, Thankful, Sleep)

*Notes and Homework Assignments:*_____

_____

_____

_____

_____

_____

_____

_____

_____

_____

_____

_____

_____

_____

_____

_____

_____

_____

_____

_____

*Tomorrow I will focus on:*_____

_____

_____

Su Mo Tu We Th Fr Sa   Date:_____

Last night, I went to bed at_____, I woke up at_____, I got_____ hrs of sleep

I slept: GREAT!   Good   Not so bad   Interrupted   UGH, bad

Today I felt so thankful for:_____
_____

How and when I can be active today:_____
_____

Challenges I expect to face today:_____
_____

I plan to overcome by:_____
_____

Food & Mood

Time of day	Food and Drink	I'm Feeling…….
Wake to 8am		
8am to 10am		
10am to 12pm		
12noon to 2pm		
2pm to 4pm		
4pm to 6pm		
6pm to 8pm		
8pm to 10pm		

Targets for the Day: P L A N T S

Give yourself a check for each target: ☐ ☐ ☐ ☐ ☐ ☐

(Plan ahead, Lots of healthy food, Activity, Nice, Thankful, Sleep)

Notes and Homework Assignments:_____

_____

_____

_____

_____

_____

_____

_____

_____

_____

_____

_____

_____

_____

_____

_____

_____

_____

Tomorrow I will focus on:_____

_____

_____

Su Mo Tu We Th Fr Sa   Date:_____

Last night, I went to bed at_____, I woke up at_____, I got_____ hrs of sleep

I slept: GREAT!   Good   Not so bad   Interrupted   UGH, bad

Today I felt so thankful for:_____
_____

How and when I can be active today:_____
_____

Challenges I expect to face today:_____
_____

I plan to overcome by:_____
_____

Food & Mood

Time of day	Food and Drink	I'm Feeling.......
Wake to 8am		
8am to 10am		
10am to 12pm		
12noon to 2pm		
2pm to 4pm		
4pm to 6pm		
6pm to 8pm		
8pm to 10pm		

Targets for the Day: P L A N T S

Give yourself a check for each target: ☐ ☐ ☐ ☐ ☐ ☐

(Plan ahead, Lots of healthy food, Activity, Nice, Thankful, Sleep)

*Notes and Homework Assignments:*_____

_____

_____

_____

_____

_____

_____

_____

_____

_____

_____

_____

_____

_____

_____

_____

_____

_____

_____

*Tomorrow I will focus on:*_____

_____

_____

Su Mo Tu We Th Fr Sa   Date:_____

Last night, I went to bed at_____, I woke up at_____, I got_____ hrs of sleep

I slept: GREAT!   Good   Not so bad   Interrupted   UGH, bad

Today I felt so thankful for:_____
_____

How and when I can be active today:_____
_____

Challenges I expect to face today:_____
_____

I plan to overcome by:_____
_____

Food & Mood

Time of day	Food and Drink	I'm Feeling…….
Wake to 8am		
8am to 10am		
10am to 12pm		
12noon to 2pm		
2pm to 4pm		
4pm to 6pm		
6pm to 8pm		
8pm to 10pm		

Targets for the Day: P L A N T S

Give yourself a check for each target: ☐ ☐ ☐ ☐ ☐ ☐

(Plan ahead, Lots of healthy food, Activity, Nice, Thankful, Sleep)

*Notes and Homework Assignments:*_____

_____

_____

_____

_____

_____

_____

_____

_____

_____

_____

_____

_____

_____

_____

_____

_____

_____

_____

_____

_____

*Tomorrow I will focus on:*_____

_____

_____

Su Mo Tu We Th Fr Sa   Date:_____

Last night, I went to bed at_____, I woke up at_____, I got_____ hrs of sleep

I slept: GREAT!   Good   Not so bad   Interrupted   UGH, bad

Today I felt so thankful for:_____
_____

How and when I can be active today:_____
_____

Challenges I expect to face today:_____
_____

I plan to overcome by:_____
_____

Food & Mood

Time of day	Food and Drink	I'm Feeling.......
Wake to 8am		
8am to 10am		
10am to 12pm		
12noon to 2pm		
2pm to 4pm		
4pm to 6pm		
6pm to 8pm		
8pm to 10pm		

Targets for the Day: P L A N T S

Give yourself a check for each target: ☐ ☐ ☐ ☐ ☐ ☐

(Plan ahead, Lots of healthy food, Activity, Nice, Thankful, Sleep)

*Notes and Homework Assignments:*_____

_____

_____

_____

_____

_____

_____

_____

_____

_____

_____

_____

_____

_____

_____

_____

_____

_____

*Tomorrow I will focus on:*_____

_____

_____

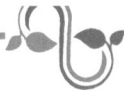

Congratulations! You've made it through the first 7 days! Let's review!

Tally the week's totals
for each target:

P L A N T S   Total   %

___ ___ ___ ___ ___ ___   ⟋42 ___

Goal: 80%

The hardest thing for me this week was:_____

_____

I found it most surprising that: _____

_____

_____

When I think about the changes I'm making in my life, I'm feeling: _____

_____

_____

I'm really struggling with:_____

_____

In order to move past this, I need to reach out for help. I can reach out to:

- _____

- _____

- _____

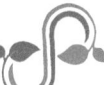

For the next week I'd like to focus on:

_____

_____

_____

_____

_____

My other thoughts / observations / goals:

_____

_____

_____

_____

_____

_____

_____

_____

You're doing great! Stick with the program, and you will continue releasing old patterns and establishing new habits. Keep at it and you will be so glad that you did!"

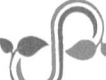

Su Mo Tu We Th Fr Sa   Date:_____

Last night, I went to bed at_____, I woke up at_____, I got____ hrs of sleep

I slept: GREAT!   Good   Not so bad   Interrupted   UGH, bad

Today I felt so thankful for:_____
_____

How and when I can be active today:_____
_____

Challenges I expect to face today:_____
_____

I plan to overcome by:_____
_____

Food & Mood

Time of day	Food and Drink	I'm Feeling.......
Wake to 8am		
8am to 10am		
10am to 12pm		
12noon to 2pm		
2pm to 4pm		
4pm to 6pm		
6pm to 8pm		
8pm to 10pm		

Targets for the Day: P L A N T S

Give yourself a check for each target: ☐ ☐ ☐ ☐ ☐ ☐

(Plan ahead, Lots of healthy food, Activity, Nice, Thankful, Sleep)

*Notes and Homework Assignments:*_____

_____

_____

_____

_____

_____

_____

_____

_____

_____

_____

_____

_____

_____

_____

_____

_____

_____

*Tomorrow I will focus on:*_____

_____

_____

Su Mo Tu We Th Fr Sa   Date:_____

Last night, I went to bed at_____, I woke up at_____, I got_____ hrs of sleep

I slept: GREAT!   Good   Not so bad   Interrupted   UGH, bad

Today I felt so thankful for:_____
_____

How and when I can be active today:_____
_____

Challenges I expect to face today:_____
_____

I plan to overcome by:_____
_____

Food & Mood

Time of day	Food and Drink	I'm Feeling.......
Wake to 8am		
8am to 10am		
10am to 12pm		
12noon to 2pm		
2pm to 4pm		
4pm to 6pm		
6pm to 8pm		
8pm to 10pm		

Targets for the Day: P L A N T S

Give yourself a check for each target: ☐ ☐ ☐ ☐ ☐ ☐

(Plan ahead, Lots of healthy food, Activity, Nice, Thankful, Sleep)

Notes and Homework Assignments:_____

_____

_____

_____

_____

_____

_____

_____

_____

_____

_____

_____

_____

_____

_____

_____

_____

_____

_____

_____

Tomorrow I will focus on:_____

_____

_____

Su Mo Tu We Th Fr Sa   Date:_____

Last night, I went to bed at_____, I woke up at_____, I got_____ hrs of sleep

I slept: GREAT!   Good   Not so bad   Interrupted   UGH, bad

Today I felt so thankful for:_____
_____

How and when I can be active today:_____
_____

Challenges I expect to face today:_____
_____

I plan to overcome by:_____
_____

Food & Mood

Time of day	Food and Drink	I'm Feeling.......
Wake to 8am		
8am to 10am		
10am to 12pm		
12noon to 2pm		
2pm to 4pm		
4pm to 6pm		
6pm to 8pm		
8pm to 10pm		

Targets for the Day: P L A N T S

Give yourself a check for each target: ☐ ☐ ☐ ☐ ☐ ☐

(Plan ahead, Lots of healthy food, Activity, Nice, Thankful, Sleep)

Notes and Homework Assignments:_____

_____

_____

_____

_____

_____

_____

_____

_____

_____

_____

_____

_____

_____

_____

_____

_____

_____

_____

_____

Tomorrow I will focus on:_____

Notes and Homework Assignments:_____

_____

Su Mo Tu We Th Fr Sa   Date:_____

Last night, I went to bed at_____, I woke up at_____, I got_____ hrs of sleep

I slept: GREAT!   Good   Not so bad   Interrupted   UGH, bad

Today I felt so thankful for:_____
_____

How and when I can be active today:_____
_____

Challenges I expect to face today:_____
_____

I plan to overcome by:_____
_____

Food & Mood

Time of day	Food and Drink	I'm Feeling.......
Wake to 8am		
8am to 10am		
10am to 12pm		
12noon to 2pm		
2pm to 4pm		
4pm to 6pm		
6pm to 8pm		
8pm to 10pm		

Targets for the Day: P L A N T S

Give yourself a check for each target: ☐ ☐ ☐ ☐ ☐ ☐

(Plan ahead, Lots of healthy food, Activity, Nice, Thankful, Sleep)

Notes and Homework Assignments:_____

_____

_____

_____

_____

_____

_____

_____

_____

_____

_____

_____

_____

_____

_____

_____

_____

_____

_____

_____

Tomorrow I will focus on:_____

_____

_____

Su Mo Tu We Th Fr Sa   Date:_____

Last night, I went to bed at_____, I woke up at_____, I got_____ hrs of sleep

I slept: GREAT!   Good   Not so bad   Interrupted   UGH, bad

Today I felt so thankful for:_____
_____

How and when I can be active today:_____
_____

Challenges I expect to face today:_____
_____

I plan to overcome by:_____
_____

Food & Mood

Time of day	Food and Drink	I'm Feeling.......
Wake to 8am		
8am to 10am		
10am to 12pm		
12noon to 2pm		
2pm to 4pm		
4pm to 6pm		
6pm to 8pm		
8pm to 10pm		

Targets for the Day: P L A N T S

Give yourself a check for each target: ☐ ☐ ☐ ☐ ☐ ☐

(Plan ahead, Lots of healthy food, Activity, Nice, Thankful, Sleep)

Notes and Homework Assignments:_____

_____

_____

_____

_____

_____

_____

_____

_____

_____

_____

_____

_____

_____

_____

_____

_____

_____

_____

Tomorrow I will focus on:_____

_____

Su Mo Tu We Th Fr Sa   Date:_____

Last night, I went to bed at_____, I woke up at_____, I got_____ hrs of sleep

I slept: GREAT!   Good   Not so bad   Interrupted   UGH, bad

Today I felt so thankful for:_____
_____

How and when I can be active today:_____
_____

Challenges I expect to face today:_____
_____

I plan to overcome by:_____
_____

Food & Mood

Time of day	Food and Drink	I'm Feeling.......
Wake to 8am		
8am to 10am		
10am to 12pm		
12noon to 2pm		
2pm to 4pm		
4pm to 6pm		
6pm to 8pm		
8pm to 10pm		

Targets for the Day: P L A N T S

Give yourself a check for each target: ☐ ☐ ☐ ☐ ☐ ☐

(Plan ahead, Lots of healthy food, Activity, Nice, Thankful, Sleep)

Notes and Homework Assignments:_____

_____

_____

_____

_____

_____

_____

_____

_____

_____

_____

_____

_____

_____

_____

_____

_____

_____

_____

Tomorrow I will focus on:_____

_____

Congratulations! You've made it through 14 days! Let's review!

Tally the week's totals
for each target:

P L A N T S   Total   %

___ ___ ___ ___ ___ ___   ⟋42 ___

Goal: 80%

The hardest thing for me this week was:_____

_____

I found it most surprising that: _____

_____

_____

When I think about the changes I'm making in my life, I'm feeling: _____

_____

_____

I'm really struggling with:_____

_____

In order to move past this, I need to reach out for help. I can reach out to:

- _____

- _____

- _____

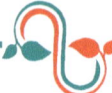

Going forward I'd like to focus on:

_____

_____

_____

_____

My other thoughts / observations / goals:

_____

_____

_____

_____

_____

_____

_____

You're doing great! Stick with the program, and you will continue releasing old patterns and establishing new habits. Keep at it and you will be so glad that you did!

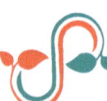